INDIAN AYURVEDA MEDICINE

ABOUT THE BOOK

This book contents the techniques of **Indian Ayurveda medicine**, it is a system of medicine with historical roots in the Indian subcontinent. Globalized and modernized practices derived from Ayurveda traditions are a type of complementary or alternative medicine. In the Western world, Ayurveda therapies and practices (which are manifold) have been integrated in general wellness applications and as well in some cases in medical use.

INDIAN AYURVEDA MEDICINE

INDIAN AYURVEDA MEDICINE

This Book Is Dedicated To My Grandmom Who Helped Me To Write This Books On Ayurveda and As An Indian It Is My Duty to Spread The Beauty of Ayurveda To The World.

1. HOME REMEDIES FOR HANGOVER

Drink plenty of water before going to bed as well as when you wake up in the morning.

Eating some foodstuff while and after you are drinking will slow down the rate at which alcohol enters the blood, thereby reducing the hangover.

Consume vitamin C tablets, as they lead to the breakdown of alcohol content in the body.

2. NATURAL AYURVEDIC HOME REMEDIES FOR ALCOHOLISM

REMEDIES FOR ALCOHOLISM

- Alcoholism is a psychological condition
- Addiction to alcohol can affect one's life
- negatively

INDIAN AYURVEDA MEDICINE

- Family support and encouragement is critical to
- help quit drinking

<u>SYMPTOMS</u>

- Depression
- Anxiety
- Irritability
- Regular absence from work
- Insomnia
- Frequent intoxicated state

<u>SIMPLE TECHNIQUES</u>

<u>method1.</u>
Natural home remedy using carom seeds
- Take 500 g of carom seeds
- Add them to 8 L of water
- Boil the mixture till about 2 L water is left
- Filter the mixture
- Drink 3-4 tbsp whenever you get a
- craving for alcohol

method2.

Natural home remedy using apple juice

- Drink 2 glasses of apple juice everyday to reduce the craving

These remedies are based on the principles of Ayurveda, the ancient Indian science of healing, and

are completely natural, non-invasive, and can be prepared at home. Consult your doctor if the symptoms persist. Refer to the terms of use.

3. ALLERGIES -
Natural Home Remedies for Allergies

- An allergic reaction occurs when the immune system reacts abnormally to certain stimuli
- Reactions to allergens vary from child to child

INDIAN AYURVEDA MEDICINE

SYMPTOMS

- Runny nose
- Chest congestion
- Sneezing
- Hives
- Rashes
- Anaphylactic attack

SIMPLE TECHNIQUES

Method1.

Natural home remedy using carrot juice,

- Beetrootnd cucumber juice
- Take 100 ml carrot juice
- Add 50 ml beetroot juice
- Add 50 ml cucumber juice
- Mix well
- Give this mixture to the child once every day. This will heal the allergic reaction and prevent it from spreading.

INDIAN AYURVEDA MEDICINE

Method2.Natural home remedy using lemon and honey

- Take 1 glass lukewarm water
- Add 4 tbsp lemon juice
- Add 1 tsp honey
- Mix well
- Let the child drink this on an empty stomach.

Tips

- Be observant & try to identify the allergens
- Most common food allergies are
- Milk
- Eggs
- Peanuts
- Soybeans
- Wheat
- Fish

- Insect bites may also trigger allergies.Get your kid diagnosed at earliest

These remedies are based on the principles of

Ayurveda, the ancient Indian science of healing, and

are completely natural, non-invasive, and can be

prepared at home. Consult your doctor if the

symptoms persist. Refer to the terms of use.

4 ALZHEIMER'S DISEASE
REMEDIES FOR ALZHEIMER'S DISEASE

- Alzheimer's is the most common form of dementia.
- Dementia is the inability of the brain to function properly due to old age.
- It is a degenerative neurological disorder.

CAUSES

- Gradual fall in level of neurotransmitters in the brain, which are responsible for transmitting messages in the brain

INDIAN AYURVEDA MEDICINE

- Presence of abnormal protein bundles in brain which leads to loss of connection between the brain cells

SYMPTOMS

1. Difficulty in recognizing known people or things Inability to remember recent activities or events

2. Forgetting common words while speaking, reading or writing

3. Inability to do routine chores like bathing, grooming or eating

4. Highly emotional behaviour

5. Depression and anxiety

SIMPLE TECHNIQUES

Method1.

Natural home remedy using almonds

1. Soak 7-8 almonds in water overnight

2. Peel off the skin in the morning

3. Eat them on an empty stomach

4. Do this for 3-4 months

method2.

Natural home remedy using lemon/

peppermint oil(To fight the lethargy and depression

caused by Alzheimer's)

1. Take the juice of half a lemon or 5-10

2. drops of peppermint oil

3. Add it to a bowl of hot water

4. Inhale the fumes

method3.Natural home remedy using sesame oil

1. Put 3 drops of sesame oil in each nostril.

2. Do this twice a day.

3. Lukewarm sesame oil can also be.

4. applied on head and feet of the patient.

5. REMEDIES FOR AMNESIA

REMEDIES FOR AMNESIA

Amnesia refers to partial or a total memory loss

Amnesia is of two types

• Anterograde

INDIAN AYURVEDA MEDICINE

- Retrogra

<u>CAUSES</u>

1. Accident or brain trauma

2. Age

3. Excessive alcohol

4. Illicit drugs

<u>SYMPTOMS</u>

<u>Anterograde amnesia</u>

1. Person cannot remember any new information

2. Affects short term memory

3. Patient continuously forgets events, people, information at short intervals

<u>Retrograde amnesia</u>

1. Patient can remember new events, but forgets the past

2. The patient forgets events or information from the period before the onset of the condition

<u>SIMPLE TECHNIQUES</u>

<u>Method1.</u>Natural home remedy using almonds and

butter

1. Soak 7-8 almonds in water overnight

2. Peel and crush them in the morning

3. Add 1 tsp of butter

4. Mix well

5. Eat this every morning

method 2.Natural home remedy using cumin powder

and honey

1. Take 2 tsp of cumin powder

2. Add 1 tbsp honey

3. Eat every morning

6. ANAEMIA
REMEDIES FOR ANAEMIA

1. Anaemia is a common blood disorder

2. Anaemic patients have low red blood cell count These cells are responsible for delivering oxygen from the lungs to other body parts

INDIAN AYURVEDA MEDICINE

CAUSES

1. Iron deficiency

2. Loss of blood, especially during menstruation

3. Reduced levels of erythropoietin, a hormone produced by the kidneys

SYMPTOMS

1. Weakness

2. Dizziness

3. Fatigue

4. Lack of energy

5. Premature wrinkling

6. Droopy eyes

7. Weak memory

8. Breathlessness on exertion

9. Headache

10. Slow healing

11. Hair loss

12. Palpitations

method

1. Take cold water baths 2 times every day

2. Expose yourself to the morning sun

3. Avoid tea and coffee as they hamper absorption of iron

7. WEIGHT LOSS

- Being overweight is harmful to one's self esteem
- It is also a health concern since it leads to many serious ailments including:

1) Diabetes

2) High blood pressure

CAUSES

1. Some people overeat when they are:

2. Depressed

3. Bored

4. Angry

5. In a relaxed environment

INDIAN AYURVEDA MEDICINE

a. Incorrect lifestyle

b. Improper diet

c. Lack of exercise

d. Hypothyroidism

SIMPLE TECHNIQUES

Methid1.

Natural home remedy for weight loss using black pepper powder, lemon juice and honey

1. Take 1 glass lukewarm water

2. Add 1 tsp black pepper powder

3. Add 4 tbsp lemon juice

4. Add 1 tsp honey

5. Mix well

6. Drink every day

TIPS

Exercise regularly

Cabbage is very effective in burning body fat. Consume 1 bowl of cabbage everyday

8. HEADACHE

Headache refers to any pain or discomfort in and around the head and neck

CAUSES

Chronic headache could be indicative of an underlying ailment

The other causes of headache include:

1. Stress

2. Lack of sleep

3. Physical exhaustion

SIMPLE TECHNIQUES

Method1.

Natural home remedy using green tea and lemon

1. Add a green tea bag

2. Squeeze $\frac{1}{2}$ a lemon

3. Mix well

4. Drink for instant relief

   Method2.

   Natural home remedy using lemon rind

1. Separate the rind (outer covering) of 2-3 lemons

2. Chop and crush the lemon rind to make a paste

3. Apply on the forehead for quick relief

   Method3.

   Natural home remedy using watermelon

   and sugar

1. Take 2 tbsp of cinnamon powder

2. Add water to make paste

3. Mix well

4. Apply on the temple and forehead for relief

   Tips:For chronic headaches:

1. Drink water mixed with honey every morning

2. Drink this on an empty stomach

9. OSTEOARTHRITIS

OSTEOARTHRITIS

1. Arthritis affects the joints causing severe pain

2. This pain can make a person immobile

3. It is one of the most common joint disorders which occurs with age

CAUSES

1. Wear and tear of the cartilage, a cushion between the bones and joints

2. Increases the friction between the bones

3. Leads to stiffness and pain in the joints

4. Overweight

5. Injury

6. Excessive exercising

7. Hereditary factors

SYMPTOMS

1. Swelling and pain in the affected joint

2. Cracking noise on any joint movement

3. Constant stiffness

Method1.Natural home remedy using potato

INDIAN AYURVEDA MEDICINE

1. Wash and cut an unpeeled potato into thin slices

2. Soak them in water overnight

3. Strain the water in the morning

4. Drink it first thing in the morning on an empty stomach

   Method2.Natural home remedy using mustard oil and

   camphor

1. Heat 1 cup of mustard oil

2. Add 10 g of camphor

3. Heat till camphor dissolves completely

4. Massage with the oil when

5. lukewarmThis increases the blood

   supply and reduces inflammation and stiffness

   Method3.

   Natural home remedy using sesame seeds

1. Take 100 ml of water

2. Soak 1 tsp of black sesame seeds in it overnight

3.Consume this mixture in the morning

method4.Natural home remedy using cinnamon powder and honey

1. Take 1 tsp of cinnamon powder

2. Add 1 tbsp of honey

3.Mix well

4.Have this on an empty stomach every morning

10. ARTHRITIS

1. Arthritis refers to severe joint pain

2.It's an auto-immune disease

3. The pain in the joints can make a person immobile

CAUSES

1. Body's tissues are attacked by their own immune system

2.Common in people over 40 years of age

SYMPTOMS

INDIAN AYURVEDA MEDICINE

- Pain and swelling in joints like:

- Fingers

- Legs

- Arms

- Wrists

- This pain is most severe in the morning

  ## SIMPLE TECHNIQUES

  Method1.

  Natural home remedy using mustard oil and camphor

1. Take 1 cup mustard oil

2. Add 10 g camphor

3. Heat the oil till the camphor dissolves completely

4. Massage lukewarm oil on the affected areaThis will help improve the blood

5. circulation in the area and will reduce the inflammation and stiffness.

   method2.

   Natural home remedy using potato

INDIAN AYURVEDA MEDICINE

1. Take a few unpeeled potato slices .

2. Soak in 1 glass cold water overnight.

3. Drink this water on an empty stomach, every morning.

   method3.

   Natural home remedy using green gram and garlic cloves

1. Take 3 tbsp green gram

2. Soak in 250 ml water overnight to get sprouted gram

3. Add 2 crushed garlic cloves to the sprouted gram 3.

4. Mix well

5. Consume 2 times a day You may add salt and pepper for taste.

11 .REMEDIES FOR ASCITES

Ascites is the accumulation of excess fluid in the abdominal area

CAUSES

INDIAN AYURVEDA MEDICINE

1. Cirrhosis of liver

2. Increased pressure of liver blood flow

SYMPTOMS

- Swelling of the abdomen

- As condition worsens one experiences

- Abdominal pain

- Discomfort

- Bloating

- There is an increase in pressure on the diaphragm, causing shortness of breath

SIMPLE TECHNIQUES

method1.

Natural home remedy using bitter gourds

1. Wash and remove the skin of 3-4 bitter gourds

2. De-seed it and crush the bitter gourds

3. Place the paste on a sieve and extract

4. the juice

5. Mix equal quantity of water

6. Drink 3 times a day

   method2.

   Natural home remedy using fenugreek seeds

1. Soak 3 tbsp fenugreek seeds overnight in 1 cup of water

2. Strain the water in the morning

   Drink on an empty stomach

   method3. Natural home remedy using chickpeas

1. Soak 1 cup of chickpeas overnight in water

2. Consume these the next day

3. Add salt and pepper to taste

12. ASTHMA

- Asthma is a condition in which the air passages in the lungs suddenly contract

- This reduces amount of air that can pass, making breathing difficult

INDIAN AYURVEDA MEDICINE

CAUSES

- Allergic asthma is a result of body's reaction to
- allergens like
- Causes of Non allergic asthma
- Dust
- Smoke
- Drugs
- Pollution
- Fear
- Anxiety
- Stress
- Excessive consumption of processed food
- High salt intake
- Low intake of omega 3 fatty acids and anti oxidants
- Genetic factors

SYMPTOMS

- Breathlessness

INDIAN AYURVEDA MEDICINE

- Pressure in the chest
- Cough

<u>SIMPLE TECHNIQUES</u>

<u>Method 1.</u>

Natural home remedy using honey

1. Fill a saucer with honey
2. Hold it beneath the nose and inhale
3. This helps to ease the breathing

Method2.

Natural home remedy using fenugreek seeds, ginger and honey

1. Take 2 tbsp of fenugreek seeds
2. Mix in 1 L of water
3. Let it simmer for 30 min
4. Strain the liquid
5. Crush ginger to make 2 tsp of ginger paste
6. Press the paste on a sieve and extract juice
7. Add ginger juice to the strained liquid

8.Add 1 tsp of honey

9. Mix well

10.   Drink 1 glass of the mixture every morning

Method3.

Natural home remedy using Indian gooseberry powder and honey

1. Take 2 tsp of Indian gooseberry powder

2.You may de-seed and crush 1 Indian

3.gooseberry and use it in place of the powder

4.Mix 1 tsp of honey

5.Have this once every morning

Tips

1. Breathe in clean air

2.Wear a cloth mask

3.Stay away from identified allergens

4.Avoid pets which have feathers or fur

13. BAD BREATH

- Bad breath can be an embarrassing condition
- It generally results from a lack of or poor oral hygiene

CAUSES

1. Bacterial activity in mouth

2. Improper oral hygiene

3. Dry mouth

4. Digestive disorders

5. Chewing tobacco

6. Consuming garlic

SYMPTOMS

1. Unpleasant odour in breath

2. Dry mouth

3. Bad taste

4. Feeling of a coating on tongue

SIMPLE TECHNIQUES

Method1.

INDIAN AYURVEDA MEDICINE

Natural home remedy using cinnamon

1. Take 1 cup of hot water

2. Add 3 tsp of cinnamon powder

3. Mix well

4. When lukewarm, use as a mouthwash

Method2.

Natural home remedy using parsley leaves

Parsley leaves are rich in chlorophyll

1. and are nature's own deodorizer.

2. Chew a few parsley leaves

Tips

1. Chew 2 cardamom seeds

2. Suck on a piece of clove after each meal

3. Eat apple or guava after each meal as it clears the food particles stuck between the teeth and prevents bacterial activity

4. Brush 2 times a day

14. REMEDIES FOR ALOPECIA

Alopecia is a condition in which the immune system starts attacking the hair follicles.

CAUSES

Genetics

1. Inflammation
2. Emotional stress
3. Excessive hair styling.
4. Poor nutrition
5. Certain medications
6. Chemotherapy
7. Hormonal changes during pregnancy or
8. menopause
9. Improper functioning of the thyroid gland
10. Scalp infections

SYMPTOMS

1. Extensive hair loss
2. Bald patches

3. Thinning hair

4. Permanent baldness

SIMPLE TECHNIQUES

Natural home remedy using essential oils

1. Take 50 ml of rose water in a glass bottle.

2. Add to it 50 ml of distilled water and

3. shake well to mix them both.

4. Now add to it 15 ml of apple cider vinegar.

5. Then add 5 drops of rosemary essential oil.

6. Also add 6 drops of jojoba oil.

7. Also put in 3 drops of carrot essential oil.

8. And then 3 drops of geranium essential oil.

9. Then close the bottle firmly and shake

10. well to mix the ingredients.

method2.

Natural home remedy using coconut and hibiscus oil

1. Crush 5 hibiscus flowers completely in a bowl.

2.Add to it ¼ cup of pure coconut oil.

3. Now mix the ingredients till they make a

4.fine paste.

5. Then apply this paste onto slightly

6.damp scalp and hair.

7.Leave it on for 2 hours and then rinse off gently with cool water and a mild shampoo.

Tips

- Handle your hair gently

- Eat iron rich food

- Exercise regularly

15. REMEDIES FOR BED WETTING

- Bed-wetting is a condition when a person unintentionally urinates while sleeping

- It is highly common amongst kids between the age of 3-5 years

- However, it can affect people of any age

SYMPTOMS

INDIAN AYURVEDA MEDICINE

- Children have an immature nervous system. It
- does not alert them when their bladder is full Small bladder is unable to retain urine produced at night
- Medical conditions like
- Urinary tract infection
- Constipation
- Diabetes
- Anaemia
- Epilepsy

SIMPLE TECHNIQUES

method1.

Natural home remedy using Indian

gooseberries, turmeric powder and honey

1. Cut, de-seed and crush 2 Indian gooseberries
2. Add a pinch of turmeric powder
3. Add 1 tsp honey
4. Mix well
5. Have 1 tsp of the mixture in the morning

INDIAN AYURVEDA MEDICINE

method2.

Natural home remedy using milk, fennel

seeds and sugar

1. Take 1 glass warm milk

2. Add 1 tsp fennel seeds

3. Take 4 tbsp of sugar

4. Add 1 glass of water to this sugar

5. Heat this mixture till it becomes a thick

6. syrup

7. Add 2 tbsp of this sugar syrup to the milk

8. Mix well

9. Drink this everyday

Tips

- Eat 2-3 walnuts and about 8-10 raisins at bedtime

- For children:

  - Avoid giving them liquids at bedtime

  - Make it a habit to urinate before

  - sleeping

16. DRY CAUGH

A dry cough is a cough that is accompanied with phlegm or mucous. Most dry coughs are a reaction to an environmental allergen, pollutant or toxin. The body attempts to expel the irritant from the respiratory system by coughing itout. A dry cough can also be a symptom ofan illness or a side effect of certain medications. In the absence of a serious illness or when medications are not the cause, home remedies can be used for treatment. Natural home treatments can reduce the frequency of coughing and cansoothe throat soreness and irritation.

Method1.

1. Drink water often to add moisture to your throat. You can drink other drinks besides water if you choose, as long as they are not acidic. Acidic drinks, such as orange juice, can irritate a dry throat.Step 2Run a humidifier in your home or office to add moisture to the air in your environment.

2. Run a humidifier in your home or office to add moisture to the air in your environment.

INDIAN AYURVEDA MEDICINE

What poison ivy looks like

Each leaf has 3 small leaflets.

It grows as a shrub (low woody plant) in the far Northern and Western United States, Canada, andaround the Great Lakes.

It grows as a vine in the East, Midwest, and South of the United States.

In spring, it grows yellow-green flowers.

It may have green berries that turn off-white in early fall.

Symptoms

- You have trouble breathing or swallowing.
- The rash covers most of yourbody.
- You have many rashes or blisters.
- You experience swelling, especially if an eyelid swells shut.
- The rash develops anywhere on your face or genitals.

- Much of your skin itches, or nothing seems to ease the itch.

SIMPLE TECHNIQUES

Method 1.

Baking Soda Baths & Pastes

Found in most kitchens, common baking soda is a great natural remedy for the itchiness associated with a poison ivy rash. To help relieve itching, place 1/2 acup of baking soda in a bath tub filled with warm water. You can also mix 3 teaspoons of baking soda with one teaspoon of water and mix until it forms a paste. Apply this paste to the infected area to relieve itching and irritation that's associated with a poison ivy rash.

Method2.

Oatmeal Paste

Cook a small amount of oatmeal and apply it directly to the skin as a paste. Make sure to cook it very thick so that the paste will stick tothe skin. Some sources recommend putting the oatmeal on the skin while it is very warm, as the heat from the oatmeal will eventually cool, leaving the skin dry and relieved. Make sure not toapply the oatmeal when it is too hot, as this can easily burn the skin. You may also try mixing in a teaspoon of baking soda, for an extra itch-relieving effect.

Method 3.

Organic Apple Cider Vinegar

Apply a teaspoon of organic applecider vinegar directly to the infected skin.Apple Cider Vinegarhas a toxin-pulling action that helps suck the poison out of the pores. You can also create a warm vinegar compress using a thin cotton towel. Reapply to the skin as needed.

method4.

Aloe Vera Gel

An ancient curative remedy for the skin, aloe vera can be used directly on the infected area. You can buy a high-quality organic version at most health-food stores, or even better, buy a plant and use the gel from inner flesh ofthe leaves. External use oforganic aloe verajuicemay also help, but is not as effective as the gel.

18. POISON OAK

INDIAN AYURVEDA MEDICINE

What poison oak looks like:

1. Each leaf has 3 small leaflets.

2. It most often grows as a shrub.

3. It can grow as a vine in the Western United States.

4. It may have yellow-white berries.

Symptoms

1. Difficulty Breathing

2. Trouble swallowing

3. Eye or facial swelling

4. Rash On Your Face, Lips, Eyes, Or Genitals

5. Rash that covers more than 25 percent of your body

6. Signs of infection, such as pus or yellow fluid leaking from blisters, or blisters that have an odor

7. Fever

8. Headache

9. Nausea

10. Swollen lymph nodes

SIMPLE TECHNIQUES

Method 1.

Baking Soda Baths & Pastes

Found in most kitchens, common baking soda is a great natural remedy for the itchiness associated with a poison oak rash. To help relieve itching, place 1/2 acup of baking soda in a bath tub filled with warm water. You can also mix 3 teaspoons of baking soda with one teaspoon of water and mix until it forms a paste. Apply this paste to the infected area to relieve itching and irritation that's associated with a poison oak rash.

Method2.

Oatmeal Paste

Cook a small amount of oatmeal and apply it directly to the skin as a paste. Make sure to cook it very thick so that the paste will stick tothe skin. Some sources recommend putting the oatmeal on the skin while it is very warm, as the heat from the oatmeal will eventually cool, leaving the skin dry and relieved. Make sure not toapply the oatmeal when it is too hot, as this can easily burn the skin. You may also try mixing in a teaspoon of baking soda, for an extra itch-relieving effect.

Method 3.

Organic Apple Cider Vinegar

Apply a teaspoon of organic applecider vinegar directly to the infected skin.Apple Cider Vinegarhas a toxin-pulling action that helps suck the poison out of the pores. You can also create a warm vinegar compress using a thin cotton towel. Reapply to the skin as needed.

method4.

Aloe Vera Gel

An ancient curative remedy for the skin, aloe vera can be used directly on the infected area. You can buy a high-quality organic version at most health-food stores, or even better, buy a plant and use the gel from inner flesh ofthe leaves. External use oforganic aloe verajuicemay also help, but is not as effective as the gel.

19. HOME REMEDIES FOR GASTRITIS

causes:-

Alcohol

- Viral and bacterial infections
- Peptic ulcer disease
- Pernicious Anemia
- High intake of spicy foods

Symptoms:-

- Abdominal bloating (tenderness and swelling [distention])
- Abdominal pain (indigestion or dyspepsia), often described as burning or gnawing
- Belching (burping)
- Dark stools
- Loss of appetite
- Nausea
- Vomiting

Methods:-

INDIAN AYURVEDA MEDICINE

1. Coconut water is just apt for treating the problem of gastritis. It gives rest to thebelly and also contains loads of vitamins and minerals. When you have gastritis, consume nothing else but coconut water throughout the day.

2. Extract the juice of potatoand drink about half cup of the juice 2-3 times everyday, but it should be consumed half an hour before meals.

3. The herb marigold is considered valuable in treating gastritis. Consume1 tbsp of this herb two times in a day.

20. HOME REMEDIES FOR HAIR LOSS

methods:-

One of the best home remedies for treating hair loss is to massage your scalp with fingers gently. It will also aid in increasing blood circulation and lend glow to your hair.

Amla oil serves as an excellent tonic for hair conditioning. To prepare amla oil, put some dry pieces of amla in coconut oil and bring to a boil. Apply this oil on the scalp and see the wonderful results.

INDIAN AYURVEDA MEDICINE

For nourishing your hair, apply coconut milk all over your scalp and massage it into the hair roots.

1 .ACNE

REMEDIES FOR ACNE

* Acne affects 60% of youngsters between 12 to 24 years of age

* It causes embarrassment, depression and lack of confidence

CAUSES

• The body is unable to remove toxins through excretion leading to contamination of the bloodstream.

• This can be due to

1. Constipation

2. Irregular bowel movement

3. Irregular meal timings

Excess starch, sugar, oil and fat consumption

INDIAN AYURVEDA MEDICINE

<u>SYMPTOMS</u>

- Whiteheads
- Blackheads
- Pimples
- Red and itchy rashes

1.Natural home remedy using garlic

- Take 2-3 garlic cloves Crush them to make a paste
- Apply this paste on the affected parts

of the skin

- For sensitive skin, mix yogurt in the garlic paste before applying

2.Natural home remedy using garlic

- Consume three cloves of garlic everyday

for 1 month

INDIAN AYURVEDA MEDICINE

- Natural home remedy using coriander leaves and turmeric powder

3. Take a handful of washed coriander leaves

1. Crush them finely

2. Place the paste on a sieve and press to extract the juice

3. Add a pinch of turmeric powder

4. Mix well

5. Apply this mixture on the face every

night

Tips

- Drink ample water

- Include lots of fruits and vegetable in your diet

- Cleanse and exfoliate your face regularly

ACNE SCARS

Popping or scratching acne can leave scars

SIMPLE TECHNIQUES

INDIAN AYURVEDA MEDICINE

method1.

<u>Natural home remedy using aloevera</u>

- Take an aloe vera leaf
- Peel the outer green covering
- Extract the gel from inside
- Apply the gel 2 times a day
- Leave it for 30 minutes
- Wash it off

<u>Method 2</u>

- Natural home remedy using honey, lemon

Juice, almond oil and milk

- Take 1 tbsp of honey
- Add 1 tbsp lemon juice
- Add 1 tbsp almond oil
- Add 2 tbsp of milk
- Mix Well

INDIAN AYURVEDA MEDICINE

- Apply on the affected area

These remedies are based on the principles of Ayurveda, the ancient Indian science of healing, and

are completely natural, non-invasive, and can be prepared at home. Consult your doctor if the symptoms persist. Refer to the terms of use.

....The End..

Please

LeaveaReview

INDIAN AYURVEDA MEDICINE

Subhash kumar choudhary, born at Bihar in Madhubani district.He is graduated from L.N.M.U Darbhanga(Bihar). He also persuing Chartered Accoutancy course from The ICAI. He wrote so many books on poems and other interested topics and loves to write books on different subjects such as cooking, stories etc.